Low Carb Slow Cooker

Easy Crock-Pot Dump Meal Recipes

Sarah Spencer

ISBN: 978-1530529520

ISBN-10:1530529522

Printed in the United States

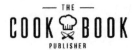

Avant-Propos

Have you committed yourself to healthy, low carb living? The type of low carb living that does not involve an overabundance of heavy meats and fats, but instead a focus on the proper portions of proteins, combined with nutritionally dense vegetables that eliminates the bad, processed carbs? The balance of a healthy protein-to-carbohydrate ratio is important for long term success and health with this type of dietary lifestyle. Perhaps you are new to low carb living, or maybe you have been savoring the benefits for years, but either way, there is a good chance that you are looking for a little variety, not only in flavors and textures, but also in the way you prepare the foods.

This is where low carbohydrate slow cooking can make a difference in your life. No longer will you be held back by your lack of time and energy towards the end of the day. All you need for most of these meals is ten to fifteen minutes to prepare the ingredients and one of the most cherished kitchen devices — the slow cooker. Slow cooking encourages healthy, homemade meals that simmer and cook all day to develop rich flavors without the need for excess fats or ingredients that could potentially sabotage your eating lifestyle. This book shows you how to bring new and exciting flavors to life, and how to have them ready for you, your friends, and family with little effort. Now is the time to recommit to your health, and the health of those that you care about.

Open up your cupboard, reach into the back and dust off the slow cooker that you thought was only for Sunday chili and an occasional roast. Your slow cooker offers you an entrance into an exciting and satisfying culinary world.

Contents

Introduction

What are the images that come to mind when you think of low carb eating? Do you envision only a limited variety of meats, cheese, and maybe a couple of vegetables prepared only a couple of simple ways? If this is you, then you are not alone. It is a common misconception about low carb dietary lifestyles that they are boring and offer little variety. Then, in addition to that, there is the issue of time. Who has time to prepare and cook dishes that are heavy in protein every single day? This, again, is another common misconception of low carb eating. The truth is that low carb eating isn't as much about what you are taking out of your diet as it about adding the right things in. One of the ways you can eat healthy low carb food every day is by bringing your slow cooker in as the star of the show.

Low carb diets have been popular for a couple of decades now. The trends have come and gone, and the dietary approach itself has evolved over time. Low carb eating is about so much more than rapid weight loss. Low carb eating is actually a lifestyle approach to overall health, weight loss, and weight maintenance. Low carbohydrate living is a focus on ingredients that are healthy and fresh, not heavy with saturated fats. Although rich, nutty, and delicious cheeses certainly have their place, as do other dairy products and red meats, these are foods that you can enjoy occasionally rather than shy away from. But more importantly, low carbohydrate living is about inclusion, rather than exclusion. The inclusion of fresh, fiber and nutrient rich vegetables and even fruits that promote and encourage

1

good health. When your carbohydrates and protein are in balance in the proper amounts you will receive health benefits that include weight loss, blood sugar regulation, reduction in inflammation, and a decreased risk of serious health issues such as heart disease, and diabetes. What's more is that you really do not even need a special diet plan. All you need instead is the understanding that processed carbohydrates are bad, like the ones found in most pre-packaged foods, including common breads, pastas, and cereals, and that naturally occurring carbohydrates in fresh foods are good.

You may have heard when starting out on a low carb dietary plan that you should severely limit your carbohydrate intake for a couple of weeks, and slowly build your intake up. This will result in rapid weight loss, mostly in the form of water, and it is completely up to you if you choose this approach. However, if you are simply looking to regain your health, feel better, or drop weight in a quicker than usual manner, then the recipes in this book, and others like them, will help you achieve your goals and show you how you can incorporate a variety of foods, many of them you may have thought were forbidden, into your diet.

With the use of a slow cooker, you will find it is possible to combine unique flavors with some of your favorite standby ingredients. The major benefit of slow cooker preparation is the way that it eases not only the budget, but also your schedule. With just a few minutes earlier in the day, you can come home to a perfectly prepared and delicious meal that is ready, waiting for you with no fuss. What you will find in this book is an incredible variety of low carb dishes that have been created specifically to be prepared in your slow cooker. The ingredients are fresh with a focus on not only protein and carbohydrate count, but fiber and other nutrients that are vital to your long term health and wellbeing. In this book, you will find an emphasis on vegetables, which may be something that you do not always associate with low carb dietary lifestyles. Many vegetables are low in carbs and high enough in other nutrients that they make valuable additions to your daily diet. Each recipe in this book is formulated to contain fifteen grams or less net carbs per serving. This is the perfect limit for assuring that you allow yourself enough nutrients, while avoiding damaging and harmful processed carbohydrates — focusing on healthy choices instead.

The ideal of low carb eating is healthy, simple, and delicious. The recipes in this book show you just how to achieve that ideal with the help of one simple, common piece of kitchen equipment. So, dig your slow cooker out of the back of the cupboard because it is about to help you achieve and maintain the best health of your life.

Simple Soups and Stews

So many times, people have an image of low carb eating that includes only red meats and cheeses. Nothing could be further from the truth. In this section, we introduce you to unique, flavorful soups and stews that will make sure that you will never be stuck in a rut of low carb options. With easy preparation, these soups and stews will provide enjoyable and warming nourishment to the body and soul.

Spicy Pumpkin Chicken Soup

Cook time 4-6 hours
Prep time 10 minutes
Serves 6

Ingredients
1 pound boneless, skinless chicken breasts, cubed
1 cup yellow onion, diced
1 cup celery, diced
3 cloves garlic, crushed and minced
1 cup red bell pepper, sliced
4 cups chicken stock
2 cups pureed pumpkin
2 teaspoons tarragon
½ teaspoon cayenne powder
½ teaspoon nutmeg
1 teaspoon salt
1 teaspoon white pepper
4 cups fresh spinach, torn

Directions

1. Set up and prepare your slow cooker.
2. Add the chicken, followed by the onion, celery, garlic, and bell pepper.
3. In a bowl, combine the chicken stock, pumpkin, tarragon, cayenne powder, nutmeg, and white pepper. Mix well and add to the slow cooker. Stir gently.
4. Cover and cook for 4 hours on HIGH or 6 hours on LOW.
5. Half an hour before the end of the cooking time, open the lid and mix in the spinach. Cook until the spinach is wilted and heated through.

Nutritional information

Calories 187
Total fat 4 g, saturated fat 1 g
Net carbohydrates 12 g
Protein 23 g

Monterey Corn Chowder

Cook Time: 4-6 hours
Prep Time: 10 minutes
Serves: 6

Ingredients:

1 pound boneless skinless chicken breast, cubed
1 red onion, diced
3 cloves garlic, crushed and minced
1 tablespoon jalapeno pepper, diced
1 cup red bell pepper, diced
1 cup fresh corn kernels
1 tablespoon olive oil
4 cups chicken stock
½ cup picante sauce
1 tablespoon ground cumin
2 teaspoons cayenne sauce
2 tablespoons cornstarch
1 cup milk (2%)
1 cup Monterey jack cheese, shredded
Fresh cilantro for garnish

Directions:

1. Set up and prepare your slow cooker.
2. Add the chicken, followed by the onion, garlic, jalapeno pepper, red bell pepper, and corn kernels.
3. Add the olive oil and toss lightly to coat.
4. Combine the chicken stock, picante sauce, cumin, cayenne sauce, and cornstarch. Whisk well until no lumps remain.
5. Add the stock mixture to the slow cooker.

6. Cover and cook for 4 hours on HIGH or 6 hours on LOW.
7. About half an hour before you are ready to eat, remove the lid and add the milk or heavy cream and Monterey jack cheese. Mix in before replacing the cover and continuing to cook.
8. Serve garnished with fresh cilantro, if desired.

Nutritional information:

Calories 273

Total fat 10 g, saturated fat 5 g

Net carbohydrates 14 g

Protein 28 g

Mexican Crab Bisque

Cook Time: 2 hours
Prep Time: 10 minutes
Serves: 4-6

Ingredients:
1 pound crab meat
1 cup yellow onion, diced
3 cloves garlic, crushed and minced
2 teaspoons chili powder
1 teaspoon cumin
1 teaspoon coriander
3 cups chicken or vegetable stock
1 cup milk or heavy cream
½ cup sour cream
Cubed avocado, for garnish if desired

Directions:
1. Set up and prepare your slow cooker.
2. Add the crab meat, onion and garlic.
3. Season with the chili powder, cumin, and coriander.
4. Add the chicken or vegetable stock.
5. Cover and cook for 2 hours on LOW.
6. About half an hour before you are ready to eat, remove the lid and add the milk or heavy cream and sour cream. Mix well before replacing the lid and continuing to cook.

7. Depending upon the desired texture of the soup, you can remove half of the soup and puree it in a blender before adding it back into the slow cooker. This will give your soup more of a bisque texture as opposed to a more rustic, chunkier texture.
8. Serve garnished with fresh avocado, if desired.

Nutritional information:
Calories 300
Total fat 11 g, saturated fat 5 g
Net carbohydrates 12 g
Protein 34 g

Easy Gumbo

Cook Time: 4 hours
Prep Time: 10 minutes
Serves: 4-6

Ingredients:
½ pound boneless skinless chicken breast, cubed
½ pound smoked ham, cubed
¼ cup peppered bacon, diced and lightly browned
½ cup yellow onion, diced
½ cup celery, diced
2 cloves garlic, crushed and minced
½ cup poblano pepper, diced
1 cup frozen okra, sliced
2 cups canned crushed tomatoes, including liquid
2 cups chicken stock
1 teaspoon cayenne powder
2 teaspoons cayenne pepper sauce
1 teaspoon salt
1 teaspoon black pepper

Directions:
1. Set up and prepare your slow cooker.
2. Add the chicken, followed by the ham, bacon, onion, celery, garlic, poblano peppers, and okra.
3. Next add the crushed tomatoes, including liquid, along with the chicken stock.
4. Season with cayenne powder, cayenne pepper sauce, salt, and black pepper.
5. Cover and cook on LOW for 4 hours.

Nutritional information:
Calories 251
Total fat 7 g, saturated fat 2 g
Net carbohydrates 8 g
Protein 32 g

Garlicky Chicken Stew

Cook Time: 4-6 hours
Prep Time: 10 minutes
Serves: 8

Ingredients:
2 pounds boneless chicken, both white and dark meats
1 cup red onion, sliced
2 cups sweet potatoes, cubed
2 cups mini portabella mushrooms, halved
1 cup celery, diced
6 cloves garlic, crushed and minced
1 sprig fresh rosemary
2 bay leaves
1 teaspoon salt
1 teaspoon black pepper
4 cups chicken stock
2 tablespoons soy sauce
1 tablespoon cornstarch

Directions:
1. Set up and prepare your slow cooker.
2. Add the chicken, followed by the red onion, sweet potatoes, mini portabella mushrooms, celery, and garlic.
3. Season with the rosemary, bay leaves, salt, and black pepper.
4. In a bowl, combine the chicken stock, soy sauce, and cornstarch. Mix with a whisk until no lumps remain.
5. Add the broth to the slow cooker.
6. Cover and cook for 4 hours on HIGH or 6 hours on LOW.

Nutritional information:
Calories 130
Total fat 2 g, saturated fat 1 g
Net carbohydrates 15 g
Protein 10 g

Chili Releno Soup

Cook Time: 4-6 hours
Prep Time: 10 minutes
Serves: 4-6

Ingredients:
1 pound beef stew meat
1 cup red onion, diced
3 cups canned stewed tomatoes, with liquid
4 cloves garlic, crushed and minced
2 cups poblano peppers, seeded and chopped
2 cups beef stock
1 tablespoon chili powder
1 teaspoon cinnamon
¼ cup fresh cilantro, chopped
1 cup Cotija cheese, crumbled
Diced avocado for garnish
Additional cilantro for garnish

Directions:
1. Set up and prepare your slow cooker.
2. Add the stew meat, followed by the red onion, stewed tomatoes and liquid, garlic, and poblano peppers.
3. Combine the beef stock with the chili powder, cinnamon, and cilantro. Mix and add to the slow cooker.
4. Cover and cook for 4 hours on HIGH or 6 hours on LOW.
5. About half an hour before you are ready to eat, remove the lid and add the Cotija cheese. Mix well before replacing the cover and continuing to cook.

6. Serve garnished with avocado and fresh cilantro, if desired.

Nutritional information:

Calories 283

Total fat 11 g, saturated fat 6 g

Net carbohydrates 8 g

Protein 30 g

Three Cheese French Onion Soup

Cook Time: 4 hours
Prep Time: 15 minutes
Serves: 6

Ingredients:
6 cups sweet yellow onions, thinly sliced
1 tablespoon olive oil
1 sprig fresh rosemary
1 tablespoon fresh thyme
6 cups beef stock
½ cup Swiss cheese, shredded
½ cup Brie cheese, sliced thick
½ cup fresh grated Parmesan cheese

Directions:
1. Set up and prepare your slow cooker.
2. Add the onions, followed by the olive oil, rosemary, and thyme. Toss to mix.
3. Add the beef stock, cover and cook on LOW for 4 hours.
4. Preheat the broiler of your oven, and ladle the soup into heat proof bowls.
5. Layer on a piece of Brie cheese, followed by some Swiss and Parmesan cheese.
6. Place under the broiler for 2-3 minutes, or until cheese melts and caramelizes lightly.

Nutritional information:
Calories 207
Total fat 11 g, saturated fat 6 g
Net carbohydrates 11 g
Protein 15 g

New Chicken Favorites

Chicken is one of the favorite protein choices for the low carb lifestyle. It is lean, easy to prepare and extremely versatile, lending itself to an endless variety of dishes. In this section we have taken flavors both classic and new, and modified them to be created in just a few simple steps with your slow cooker.

Parmesan Crab Stuffed Chicken

Cook Time: 6 hours
Prep Time: 15 minutes
Serves: 4

Ingredients:

4 boneless, skinless chicken breasts, butterflied and pounded thin
½ pound crab meat
1 tablespoon shallots, chopped
1 teaspoon lemon zest
3 cups spaghetti squash (insides only)
1 teaspoon rubbed sage
1 teaspoon tarragon
1 cup chicken stock
2 tablespoons butter, diced
1 cup fresh spinach, torn
½ cup fresh grated Parmesan cheese

Directions:

1. Set up and prepare your slow cooker.
2. In a bowl, combine the crab meat, shallots, and lemon zest.
3. Spread equal amounts of the mixture in the center of each chicken breast.
4. Roll the chicken into a pinwheel and secure with cooking twine. Set aside.
5. In another bowl, combine the spaghetti squash, rubbed sage, tarragon, and butter.
6. Place the chicken into the slow cooker.
7. Arrange the spaghetti squash around and over the chicken, and pour the chicken stock around it.
8. Cover and cook for 6 hours on LOW.
9. In the final 30 minutes of cooking, stir in the spinach and Parmesan. Cook until the spinach is wilted, and the Parmesan is melted.

Nutritional information:

Calories 513
Total fat 18 g, saturated fat 8 g
Net carbohydrates 9 g
Protein 74 g

Marinated Thai Chicken

Cook Time: 4-6 hours
Prep Time: 10 minutes plus marinating time
Serves: 4

Ingredients:
1 pound boneless skinless chicken breast, sliced into strips
¼ cup soy sauce
2 teaspoons lime juice
¼ cup fresh basil, chopped
1 teaspoon fresh ginger, grated
¼ cup plain yogurt
1 cup yellow onion, sliced
2 cups assorted mushrooms, sliced
2 cups zucchini, sliced
2 cups asparagus, cut into 1-inch pieces
1 cup chicken stock
2 teaspoons sesame oil
Sesame seeds for garnish

Directions:
1. Set up and prepare your slow cooker.
2. In a bowl, combine the soy sauce, lime juice, basil, ginger, and yogurt.
3. Toss the chicken into the sauce mixture to coat. You can either place in the refrigerator to marinate for up to 8 hours, or you can immediately add the chicken to the slow cooker and proceed with the recipe instructions.
4. Add the onion, mushrooms, zucchini, and asparagus.

5. Combine the chicken stock with the sesame oil and add to the slow cooker.
6. Cover and cook for 4 hours on HIGH, or 6 hours on LOW.
7. Serve garnished with sesame seeds, if desired.

Nutritional information:
Calories 263
Total fat 7 g, saturated fat 2 g
Net carbohydrates 11 g
Protein 33 g

Cranberry Chicken

Cook Time: 6 hours
Prep Time: 10 minutes
Serves: 6-8

Ingredients:
2 pounds bone-in chicken pieces, skins removed
3 cups sweet potatoes, cubed
1 cup cranberries
1 tablespoon shallots
½ cup celery, diced
½ cup walnuts, chopped
½ cup apple cider
½ cup chicken stock
1 tablespoon apple cider vinegar
1 teaspoon stone ground mustard
1 teaspoon cinnamon
½ teaspoon ground cloves

Directions:
1. Set up and prepare your slow cooker.
2. Add the chicken to the slow cooker, followed by the sweet potatoes, cranberries, shallots, celery, and walnuts.
3. In a bowl, combine the apple cider, chicken stock, apple cider vinegar, mustard, cinnamon, and cloves. Pour over the chicken and vegetables.
4. Cover and cook for 6 hours on LOW.

Nutritional information:
Calories 146
Total fat 6 g, saturated fat 1 g
Net carbohydrates 13 g
Protein 8 g

Elegant Mushroom Chicken

Cook Time: 4-6 hours
Prep Time: 10 minutes
Serves: 4

Ingredients:

1 pound boneless skinless chicken breast
2 cups button mushrooms, sliced
1 cup red onion, diced
2 tablespoons olive oil
½ cup chicken stock
¼ cup semi sweet white wine
¼ cup heavy cream
2 teaspoons ground sage
1 teaspoon thyme
1 teaspoon salt
1 teaspoon pepper
Fresh salad greens or zucchini noodles for serving

Directions:

1. Set up and prepare your slow cooker.
2. Add the chicken to the slow cooker, followed by the mushrooms, red onion, and olive oil. Toss to mix.
3. In a bowl, combine the chicken stock, white wine, heavy cream, ground sage, thyme, salt, and pepper. Mix well and add to the slow cooker.
4. Cover and cook for 4 hours on HIGH or 6 hours on LOW.
5. Serve with fresh salad greens or zucchini noodles.

Nutritional information:
Calories 292
Total fat 16 g, saturated fat 5 g
Net carbohydrates 5 g
Protein 28 g

Maple Balsamic Chicken

Cook Time: 6 hours
Prep Time: 10 minutes
Serves: 6

Ingredients:

2 pounds bone-in chicken pieces, skins removed
1 tablespoon olive oil
1 cup red onion, sliced
2 cups acorn squash, peeled and sliced
2 cups fresh green beans, trimmed
2 cloves garlic, crushed and minced
1 cup chicken stock
¼ cup balsamic vinegar
1 tablespoon maple syrup
¼ cup fresh basil, chopped
1 tablespoon fresh thyme, chopped
1 teaspoon salt
1 teaspoon coarse ground black pepper
¼ cup goat cheese

Directions:

1. Set up and prepare your slow cooker.
2. Place the chicken and the olive oil to the slow cooker. Toss to coat.
3. Add the red onion, acorn squash, green beans, and garlic.
4. In a bowl, combine the chicken stock, balsamic vinegar, and maple syrup. Mix well and add to the slow cooker.
5. Season with the basil, thyme, salt, and black pepper.

6. Cover and cook for 6 hours on LOW.
7. About half an hour before you are ready to eat, remove the lid and gently stir in the goat cheese. Replace the cover and continue to cook.

Nutritional information:

Calories 172
Total fat 8 g, saturated fat 2 g
Net carbohydrates 12 g
Protein 11 g

Lemongrass Chicken with Zucchini Noodles

Cook Time: 4 hours
Prep Time: 15 minutes
Serves: 4

Ingredients:
1 pound boneless skinless chicken breast, sliced into strips
1 tablespoon olive oil
½ cup ponzu or soy sauce
2 teaspoons fresh ginger, grated
2 cloves garlic, crushed and minced
1 tablespoon fresh lemongrass, chopped
1 tablespoon crushed red pepper flakes
4 cups zucchini noodles (fresh zucchini sliced into thin, noodle-like strips)
1 cup carrots, peeled and thinly sliced
2 teaspoons sesame oil
1 teaspoon black pepper
1 cup coconut milk
Chopped peanuts for garnish, if desired

Directions:
1. Set up and prepare your slow cooker.
2. Arrange the chicken strips in the slow cooker.
3. In a bowl, combine the olive oil, ponzu or soy sauce, ginger, garlic, lemongrass, and crushed red pepper flakes. Mix well and pour over the chicken.
4. Next add the zucchini noodles and carrots.
5. Season with sesame oil and black pepper.

6. Add the coconut milk, and then cover and cook for 4 hours on LOW.
7. Serve garnished with chopped peanuts, if desired.

Nutritional information:

Calories 341

Total fat 19 g, saturated fat 11 g

Net carbohydrates 10 g

Protein 29 g

Smothered Chicken

Cook Time: 6 hours
Prep Time: 10 minutes
Serves: 6

Ingredients:

1 pound boneless skinless chicken breasts
1 cup sweet yellow onion, sliced
2 cups cremini mushrooms, halved
2 cups butternut squash, peeled and cubed
2 cloves garlic, crushed and minced
1 teaspoon ground sage
1 teaspoon thyme
½ teaspoon nutmeg
1 teaspoon salt
1 teaspoon black pepper
1 cup chicken stock
½ cup heavy cream
½ cup cream cheese, cubed
½ cup Swiss cheese, shredded
¼ cup chives, chopped

Directions:
1. Set up and prepare your slow cooker.
2. Add the chicken to the slow cooker followed by the onion, cremini mushrooms, butternut squash, and garlic.
3. Season with the ground sage, thyme, nutmeg, salt, and black pepper.
4. Add the chicken stock and cover to cook for 6 hours on LOW.
5. About half an hour before you are ready to eat, add the heavy cream, cream cheese, Swiss

cheese, and chives. Mix before replacing the lid and continuing to cook.

Nutritional information:

Calories 318

Total fat 19 g, saturated fat 11 g

Net carbohydrates 11 g

Protein 24 g

Jerk Chicken with Greens

Cook Time: 6 hours
Prep Time: 10 minutes
Serves: 8

Ingredients:
2 pounds bone-in chicken pieces, skin removed
1 teaspoon cinnamon
½ teaspoon nutmeg
¼ teaspoon ground cloves
1 teaspoon salt
1 teaspoon black pepper
1 cup sweet yellow onion, sliced
3 cloves garlic, crushed and minced
2 cups sweet potatoes, cubed
4 cups fresh greens, such as collard greens
1 cup fresh pineapple chunks
1 tablespoon jalapeno pepper, diced
1 cup chicken stock
½ cup unsweetened apple juice
1 teaspoon lime juice

Directions:
1. Set up and prepare your slow cooker.
2. Add the chicken and season with cinnamon, nutmeg, cloves, salt, and black pepper.
3. Next, add the onion, garlic, sweet potatoes, pineapple chunks, and jalapeno pepper.
4. Cover with chicken stock, apple juice, and lime juice.
5. Cover and cook for 6 hours on LOW.

6. About half an hour before you are ready to eat, add the greens and stir to mix. Serve when wilted and warmed through.

Nutritional information:
Calories 115
Total fat 1 g, saturated fat 0 g
Net carbohydrates 14 g
Protein 8 g

Chicken Fajita Casserole

Cook Time: 4 hours
Prep Time: 10 minutes
Serves: 4-6

Ingredients:
1 pound boneless skinless chicken breast, cut into strips
2 teaspoons cumin
2 cloves garlic, crushed and minced
1 cup red onion, sliced
4 cups cauliflower florets
1 cup green bell pepper, sliced
1 cup red bell pepper, sliced
1 cup tomatoes, diced
1 ½ cups chicken stock
1 teaspoon chili powder
1 teaspoon paprika
½ teaspoon cinnamon
1 teaspoon salt
1 teaspoon black pepper
2 teaspoons lime juice
1 cup Cotija cheese, crumbled
½ cup cream cheese, cubed
Avocado for garnish if desired, sliced

Directions:
1. Set up and prepare your slow cooker.
2. Add the chicken breast and season with cumin before adding the garlic, red onion, cauliflower, green bell pepper, red bell pepper, and tomatoes.
3. Combine the chicken stock with the chili powder, paprika, cinnamon, salt, black pepper, and lime juice. Add to the slow cooker.

4. Cover and cook for 4 hours on LOW.
5. About half an hour before you are ready to eat, remove the lid and add the Cotija cheese and cream cheese. Mix well before replacing the lid and continuing to cook.
6. Serve garnished with fresh avocado, if desired.

Nutritional information:

Calories 491
Total fat 29 g, saturated fat 16 g
Net carbohydrates 14 g
Protein 45 g

Olive Chicken

Cook Time: 6 hours
Prep Time: 10 minutes
Serves: 4-6

Ingredients:

2 pounds bone-in chicken pieces, skin removed
1 cup pearl onions, peeled
3 cloves garlic, crushed and minced
2 cups carrots, peeled and sliced
3 cups Brussels sprouts, halved
1 cup large green olives, pitted and halved
½ cup dry white wine
1 cup chicken stock
2 sprigs fresh rosemary
1 tablespoon fresh oregano
1 teaspoon salt
1 teaspoon black pepper

Directions:

1. Set up and prepare the slow cooker.
2. Arrange the chicken in the slow cooker, followed by the pearl onions, garlic, carrots, Brussels sprouts, and green olives.
3. Combine the dry white wine with the chicken stock and add to the slow cooker.
4. Season with rosemary, oregano, salt, and black pepper.
5. Cover and cook for 6 hours on LOW.

Nutritional information:

Calories 252

Total fat 10 g, saturated fat 1 g

Net carbohydrates 13 g

Protein 15 g

Anise Blessed Chicken

Cook Time: 8 hours
Prep Time: 10 minutes
Serves: 4-6

Ingredients:
4-5 pound whole chicken
2 bay leaves
¼ cup fresh parsley
1 tablespoon fresh thyme
1 tablespoon caraway seeds
4 star anise
2 cups chicken stock
2 cups carrots, peeled and sliced
2 cups yellow squash, peeled and diced

Directions:
1. Set up and prepare your slow cooker.
2. Place the chicken in the slow cooker and season with bay leaves, parsley, thyme, caraway seeds, and star anise.
3. Add the chicken stock, carrots, and yellow squash.
4. Cover and cook for 8 hours on LOW.

Nutritional information:
Calories 198
Total fat 5 g, saturated fat 1 g
Net carbohydrates 10 g
Protein 25 g

Best Beef Dishes

Beef is rich and decadent, and a low carb lifestyle staple. The only problem with beef is that we tend to limit ourselves in the ways that we prepare it, and the flavors that we combine with it. With the help of your slow cooker, you can expand your flavor horizons and explore new tastes and textures with your beef dishes, such as the ones included in these recipes.

Peppery Roast with Beets and Sprouts

Cook Time: 8 hours
Prep Time: 10 minutes
Serves: 8

Ingredients:
1 3-4 pound beef roast
2 tablespoons coarse ground mustard
1 tablespoon coarse ground black pepper
3 cloves garlic, crushed and minced
1 teaspoon salt
2 cups beets, sliced
3 cups Brussels sprouts, chopped
1 tablespoon olive oil
1 tablespoon fresh mint

Directions:
1. Set up and prepare your slow cooker.
2. Season the roast with coarse ground mustard, black pepper, garlic, and salt before adding it to the slow cooker.

3. Next, add the beets and Brussels sprouts.
4. Drizzle with olive oil and season with fresh mint.
5. Cover and cook for 8 hours on LOW or until roast
    has reached desired doneness.

Nutritional information:

Calories 553
Total fat 35 g, saturated fat 3 g
Net carbohydrates 4 g
Protein 50 g

Irish Corned Beef Dinner

Cook Time: 6-8 hours
Prep Time: 10 minutes
Serves: 8

Ingredients:
1 3-4 pound beef brisket
1 tablespoon pickling spice
1 teaspoon ground caraway seeds
3 cups cabbage, chopped
2 cups carrots, peeled and sliced
2 cup turnips, peeled and sliced
3 cups beef stock
½ cup dark beer

Directions:
1. Set up and prepare your slow cooker.
2. Season the brisket with the pickling spice and caraway seeds before placing it in the slow cooker.
3. Add the cabbage, carrots, turnips, beef stock and dark beer.
4. Cover and cook for 6 hours on HIGH or 8 hours on LOW.

Nutritional information:
Calories 264
Total fat 7 g, saturated fat 2 g
Net carbohydrates 6 g
Protein 40 g

Cajun Beef Tips

Cook Time: 4-6 hours
Prep Time: 10 minutes
Serves: 6

Ingredients:
2 pounds sirloin beef tips
1 cup celery, diced
1 cup red onion, sliced
1 cup red bell pepper, sliced
2 cloves garlic, crushed and minced
½ cup poblano pepper, diced
2 cups canned stewed tomatoes
1 cup beef stock
2 tablespoons Cajun seasoning
1 teaspoon salt
1 teaspoon black pepper

Directions:
1. Set up and prepare your slow cooker.
2. Add the beef tips, followed by the celery, red onion, red bell pepper, garlic, poblano pepper, and stewed tomatoes.
3. Add the beef stock and Cajun seasoning, salt, and black pepper.
4. Cover and cook for 4 hours on HIGH or 6 hours on LOW.

Nutritional information:
Calories 394
Total fat 24 g, saturated fat 9 g
Total carbohydrates 8 g
Protein 31 g

Flank Steak Pinwheels and Squash

Cook Time: 8 hours
Prep Time: 15 minutes
Serves: 4-6

Ingredients:
1 pound beef flank steak
2 tablespoons olive oil
½ cup bacon, cooked and crumbled
2 cloves garlic, crushed and minced
1 cup tomatoes, diced
¼ cup fresh parsley, chopped
½ cup yellow onion, diced
¼ cup fresh basil, chopped
2 cups butternut squash, peeled and cubed
2 cups cremini mushrooms, halved
2 tablespoons Worcestershire sauce
1 tablespoon balsamic vinegar
1 cup beef stock
4 cups fresh spinach, torn

Directions:
1. Set up and prepare your slow cooker.
2. Arrange the flank steak in the slow cooker and drizzle with olive oil.
3. Add the bacon, garlic, tomatoes, parsley, yellow onion, basil, butternut squash, and cremini mushrooms.
4. In a bowl, combine the Worcestershire sauce, balsamic vinegar, and beef stock, and add to the slow cooker.
5. Cover and cook for 8 hours on LOW.

6. About half an hour before you are ready to eat, stir in the spinach and cook until wilted and heated through.

Nutritional information:
Calories 330
Total fat 16 g, saturated fat 5 g
Net carbohydrates 14 g
Protein 29 g

Steak with Spiced Coconut Sauce

Cook Time: 4-6 hours
Prep Time: 10 minutes
Serves: 4-6

Ingredients:

1 pound flank steak, sliced into strips
1 cup red onion, sliced
4 cups cauliflower florets
1 cup chickpeas, canned or cooked
1 tablespoon olive oil
2 cups beef stock
2 cups unsweetened coconut milk
½ cup shredded unsweetened coconut
1 tablespoon tomato paste
1 tablespoon lime juice
3 tablespoons soy sauce
4 cloves garlic, crushed and minced
1 tablespoon fresh grated ginger
1 teaspoon cinnamon
1 teaspoon coriander

Directions:

1. Set up and prepare your slow cooker.
2. Arrange the flank steak in the slow cooker, and layer on the red onion, cauliflower, chickpeas, and olive oil.
3. In a bowl, combine the beef stock, unsweetened coconut milk, shredded coconut, tomato paste, lime juice, soy sauce, garlic, ginger, cinnamon, and coriander. Mix well before adding to the slow cooker.

4. Cover and cook for 4 hours on HIGH or 6 hours on LOW.

Nutritional information:
Calories 370
Total fat 23 g, saturated fat 15 g
Net carbohydrates 15 g
Protein 22 g

Deconstructed Cabbage Rolls

Cook Time: 6 hours
Prep Time: 10 minutes
Serves: 6

Ingredients:

1 pound lean ground beef
½ cup bacon, cooked and crumbled
4 cups cabbage, sliced
1 cup yellow onion, diced
2 cups stewed tomatoes, with liquid
2 cloves garlic, crushed and minced
1 cup beef stock
¼ cup apple cider vinegar
½ teaspoon cinnamon
2 teaspoons caraway seeds
1 teaspoon salt
1 teaspoon black pepper

Directions:

1. Set up and prepare your slow cooker.
2. Add the ground beef, bacon, cabbage, yellow onion, stewed tomatoes, and garlic.
3. In a bowl, combine the beef stock, apple cider vinegar, cinnamon, caraway, salt, and black pepper. Mix well before adding to the slow cooker.
4. Cover and cook for 6 hours on LOW.

Nutritional information:

Calories 247

Total fat 16 g, saturated fat 6 g

Net carbohydrates 6 g

Protein 16 g

Poached Beef Tenderloin with Winter Vegetables

Cook Time: 8 hours
Prep Time: 10 minutes
Serves: 6

Ingredients:
2 pounds beef tenderloin roast
1 teaspoon salt
1 teaspoon black pepper
1 sprig fresh rosemary
1 tablespoon fresh thyme
3 cups beef stock
2 cups carrots, peeled and sliced thick
2 cups beets, peeled and sliced
2 cups parsnips, peeled and sliced

Directions:
1. Set up and prepare your slow cooker.
2. Arrange the beef tenderloin in the slow cooker and season with salt, black pepper, rosemary, and thyme.
3. Cover with beef stock and then add the carrots, beets, and parsnips.
4. Cover and cook on LOW for 8 hours.

Nutritional information:
Calories 466
Total fat 28 g, saturated fat 11 g
Net carbohydrates 14 g
Protein 33 g

Beef Taco Pot

Cook Time: 6 hours
Prep Time: 10 minutes
Serves: 4

Ingredients:

1 pound lean ground beef
1 cup red onion, diced
1 cup green bell pepper, diced
1 cup fresh corn kernels
1 cup tomatoes, chopped
1 cup poblano pepper, diced
½ cup black olives, sliced
1 tablespoon ground cumin
2 teaspoons chili powder
1 teaspoon garlic powder
1 teaspoon cayenne powder
1 teaspoon black pepper
1 teaspoon salt
½ cup beef stock or tomato juice
½ cup Cotija cheese, crumbled

Directions:

1. Set up and prepare your slow cooker.
2. Add the ground beef, red onion, green bell pepper, fresh corn kernels, tomatoes, poblano pepper and black olives.
3. Season with cumin, chili powder, garlic powder, cayenne powder, black pepper and salt.
4. Add the beef stock or tomato juice, cover and cook for 6 hours on LOW.

5. About half an hour before you are ready to eat remove the cover and add the Cotija cheese. Replace the lid and continue cooking.

Nutritional information:
Calories 463
Total fat 32 g, saturated fat 14 g
Net carbohydrates 14 g
Protein 29 g

Super Simple Swiss Steak

Cook Time: 4-6 hours
Prep Time: 10 minutes
Serves: 2-3

Ingredients:
1 pound sirloin steak, cubed
1 teaspoon salt
1 teaspoon black pepper
3 cloves garlic, crushed and minced
1 cup celery, chopped
1 cup carrots, chopped
1 cup yellow onion, sliced
2 cups canned tomatoes, with liquid
1 ½ cups beef stock
1 teaspoon tarragon

Directions:
1. Set up and prepare your slow cooker.
2. Season the steak with salt and black pepper, and arrange it in the slow cooker. Add the garlic, celery, carrots, yellow onion, and canned tomatoes (including liquid) to the slow cooker.
3. Cover with the beef stock and season with tarragon.
4. Cover and cook for 4 hours on HIGH or 6 hours on LOW, or until meat has reached desired doneness.

Nutritional information:

Calories 211

Total fat 5 g, saturated fat 2 g

Net carbohydrates 10 g

Protein 29 g

Beef Sausage and Peppers

Cook Time: 4-6 hours
Prep Time: 10 minutes
Serves: 4

Ingredients:

1 pound beef sausage links, cut into thick slices
1 cup yellow onion, sliced
1 cup red bell pepper, sliced
2 cups green bell pepper, sliced
1 cup cherry tomatoes, halved
1 cup beef stock
2 teaspoons tomato paste
½ cup fresh basil, chopped
1 tablespoon fresh oregano
1 teaspoon salt
1 teaspoon black pepper

Directions:

1. Set up and prepare your slow cooker.
2. Add the beef sausage to the slow cooker, followed by the yellow onion, red bell pepper, green bell pepper and cherry tomatoes.
3. In a bowl combine the beef stock, tomato paste, fresh basil, oregano, salt and black pepper.
4. Cover and cook for 4 hours on HIGH or 6 hours on LOW.

Nutritional information:

Calories 268
Total fat 20 g, saturated fat 7 g
Net carbohydrates 10 g
Protein 11 g

Perfect Pork, Veal and Lamb Dishes

When you are looking for something a little different, whether it be for company or just to expand your own dinner options, pork, veal, and lamb offer new choices in flavors and textures. There is no reason to shy away from these meats when using your slow cooker. They cook up beautifully tender, providing you with savory, delicious meals.

Herb Garden Stuffed Pork Loin

Cook Time: 8 hours
Prep Time: 15 minutes
Serves: 8

Ingredients:
3 pound pork tenderloin roast
¼ cup stone ground mustard
4 cloves garlic, crushed and minced
1 teaspoon black pepper
4 tablespoons butter
¼ cup fresh basil, chopped
¼ cup fresh chives, chopped
¼ cup fresh sage, chopped
2 cups cherry tomatoes, halved
2 cups fresh spinach
1 cup chicken or vegetable stock

Directions:

1. Prepare and set up your slow cooker.
2. Slice the tenderloin ¾ of the way through along one side and spread it open.
3. In a bowl, combine the butter, basil, chives, and sage. Mix well and spread along the inside of the pork.
4. Fold the pork back over, securing with cooking twine, if needed.
5. Season the pork with stone ground mustard, garlic, and black pepper. Place in the slow cooker.
6. Add the tomatoes, chicken or vegetable stock.
7. Cover and cook for 8 hours on LOW.
8. About half an hour before you are ready to eat, open the lid and stir in the spinach. Serve when the spinach is wilted and the meat is cooked through.

Nutritional information:

Calories 418
Total fat 20 g, saturated fat 7 g
Net carbohydrates 3 g
Protein 52 g

Garlic Lamb Shanks

Cook Time: 6-8 hours
Prep Time: 10 minutes
Serves: 4-6

Ingredients:
2 pound lamb shank
5 whole cloves garlic
1 tablespoon olive oil
1 cup carrots, peeled and diced
1 cup celery, diced
1 cup onion, diced
2 cups rutabaga, peeled and cubed
2 cups Swiss chard, torn
2 cups vegetable stock
2 teaspoons tomato paste
1 teaspoon honey
¼ cup dry red wine
¼ cup fresh parsley, chopped
1 tablespoon fresh thyme, chopped
1 tablespoon black peppercorns

Directions:
1. Set up and prepare your slow cooker.
2. Add the lamb to the slow cooker, together with the garlic cloves.
3. Drizzle with olive oil.
4. Add the carrots, celery, onion, and rutabaga.
5. In a bowl, combine the vegetable stock, tomato paste, honey, dry red wine, parsley, thyme and black peppercorns.

6. Pour the stock mixture over the lamb and vegetables.
7. Cover and cook on HIGH for 6 hours, or on LOW for 8 hours.

Nutritional information:
Calories 282
Total fat 9 g, saturated fat 3 g
Net carbohydrates 11 g
Protein 33 g

Pork Medallions with Fennel and Leek

Cook Time: 8 hours
Prep Time: 10 minutes
Serves: 6

Ingredients:

2 pounds pork medallions
3 cloves garlic, crushed and minced
1 tablespoon olive oil
1 cup vegetable or chicken stock
1 cup leeks, sliced
2 cups fennel bulbs, sliced
1 sprig fresh rosemary
1 teaspoon salt
1 teaspoon black pepper

Directions:

1. Set up and prepare your slow cooker.
2. Arrange the pork and the garlic in the slow cooker.
3. Drizzle with olive oil before adding the vegetable stock.
4. Add the leeks, fennel, rosemary, salt, and black pepper.
5. Cover and cook for 8 hours on LOW.

Nutritional information:

Calories 356
Total fat 15 g, saturated fat 4 g
Net carbohydrates 4 g
Protein 46 g

Sweet and Spicy Peachy Pork

Cook Time: 4-6 hours
Prep Time: 10 minutes
Serves: 4

Ingredients:
4 bone-in pork chops
¼ teaspoon cinnamon
¼ teaspoon cloves
1 tablespoon crushed red pepper flakes
1 cup sweet yellow onion, sliced
2 cups fresh peaches, sliced
1 cup chicken or vegetable stock
1 tablespoon lemon juice
2 tablespoons orange juice

Directions:
1. Set up and prepare your slow cooker.
2. Season the pork chops with the cinnamon, cloves, and crushed red pepper flakes before placing them in the slow cooker.
3. Add the onion and peaches.
4. In a bowl, combine the chicken or vegetable stock, lemon juice, and orange juice. Mix well and add to the slow cooker.
5. Cover and cook for 4 hours on HIGH, or 6 hours on LOW.

Nutritional information:
Calories 217
Total fat 7 g, saturated fat 3 g
Net carbohydrates 12 g
Protein 24 g

Veal Shank with Anchovy Sauce

Cook Time: 8 hours
Prep Time: 15 minutes
Serves: 6

Ingredients:
2 pounds veal shank cross cuts
1 cup onion, sliced
1 cup carrot, sliced
½ cup celery, diced
1 cup chicken or vegetable stock
½ cup dry white wine
¼ cup fresh parsley, chopped
1 tablespoon fresh thyme
1 teaspoon tomato paste
½ teaspoon salt
1 teaspoon black pepper

Sauce
2 cloves garlic, crushed and minced
1 teaspoon lemon zest
¼ cup fresh parsley, chopped
1 tablespoon anchovy, chopped
1 tablespoon olive oil

Directions:
1. Set up and prepare your slow cooker.
2. Place the veal in the slow cooker followed by the onion, carrot, and celery.
3. Add the chicken or vegetable stock, tomato paste, and the dry white wine.
4. Season with parsley, thyme, salt, and black pepper.

5. Cover and cook for 8 hours on LOW.
6. To make the sauce: Combine the garlic, lemon zest, parsley, anchovy, and olive oil in a blender or food processer. Pulse until smooth and serve on the side with the veal.

Nutritional information:
Calories 348
Total fat 10 g, saturated fat 2 g
Net carbohydrates 5 g
Protein 52 g

Chilied Spareribs

Cook Time: 8 hours
Prep Time: 10 minutes
Serves: 4

Ingredients:
2-3 pounds pork spareribs
2 tablespoons brown sugar
1 tablespoon chili powder
1 teaspoon cayenne powder
2 tablespoons paprika
1 teaspoon onion powder
1 teaspoon salt
1 teaspoon black pepper
2 cups yellow onion, sliced
½-1 cup chicken or vegetable stock

Directions:
1. Set up and prepare your slow cooker.
2. In a bowl, combine the brown sugar, chili powder, cayenne powder, paprika, onion powder, salt, and black pepper. Rub the mixture into the spareribs.
3. Place the spareribs in the slow cooker.
4. Cover with the yellow onion and add the vegetable stock.
5. Cover and cook for 8 hours on LOW.

Nutritional information:
Calories 484
Total fat 35 g, saturated fat 13 g
Net carbohydrates 7 g
Protein 34 g

Chinese Pork Ribs

Cook Time: 8 hours
Prep Time: 10 minutes
Serves: 4

Ingredients:
2-3 pounds pork spareribs
3 cloves garlic, crushed and minced
¼ cup soy sauce
2 tablespoons low sugar orange marmalade
3 tablespoons ketchup
3 cups bok choy, chopped
1 cup chicken or vegetable stock

Directions:
1. Set up and prepare your slow cooker.
2. In a bowl combine the soy sauce, orange marmalade and ketchup. Mix well and brush over the spareribs.
3. Place the spareribs in the slow cooker along with the garlic.
4. Add the chicken or vegetable stock.
5. Cover and cook for 8 hours on LOW.
6. About half an hour before you are ready to eat, open the lid and stir in the bok choy. Serve when the greens are wilted and the meat is tender.

Nutritional information:
Calories 482
Total fat 35 g, saturated fat 13 g
Net carbohydrates 6 g
Protein 35 g

Vegetable Stuffed Pork Chops

Cook Time: 8 hours
Prep Time: 15 minutes
Serves: 4

Ingredients:

4 bone-in pork chops
¼ cup yellow onion, diced
¼ cup red bell pepper, diced
½ cup fresh corn kernels
½ cup poblano pepper, diced
4 cups asparagus spears, cut into 1-inch pieces
1 cup chicken or vegetable stock
1 teaspoon cumin
1 teaspoon garlic powder
1 teaspoon salt
1 teaspoon black pepper

Directions:

1. Set up and prepare your slow cooker.
2. Cut the pork chops along the side, going about ¾ of the way into the meat.
3. In a bowl, combine the onion, red bell pepper, corn, and poblano peppers. Mix well and spoon the mixture into the center of each pork chop.
4. Season the pork chops with cumin, garlic powder, salt, and pepper before adding to the slow cooker.
5. Add the chicken or vegetable stock.
6. Cover and cook for 8 hours on LOW.
7. About half an hour before you are ready to eat, add the asparagus. Serve when the asparagus is tender and the meat is cooked through.

Nutritional information:
Calories 221
Total fat 7 g, saturated fat 3 g
Net carbohydrates 9 g
Protein 26 g

Peanut Pork

Cook Time: 4-6 hours
Prep Time: 10 minutes
Serves: 4-6

Ingredients:

1 pound pork, cut into slices
1 cup yellow onion, sliced
3 cups broccoli florets
1 cup chicken or vegetable stock
¼ cup sugar free creamy peanut butter
2 tablespoons soy sauce
1 tablespoon lemon juice
1 teaspoon chili powder
1 teaspoon salt
1 teaspoon black pepper
1 cup peanuts, chopped

Directions:

1. Set up and prepare your slow cooker.
2. Arrange the pork in the slow cooker, followed by the onion. If possible, keep the broccoli out until the final hour of cooking. Otherwise, add it as well.
3. In a bowl, combine the chicken or vegetable stock, peanut butter, soy sauce, lemon juice, chili powder, salt, and black pepper. Mix well and add to the slow cooker.
4. Add the peanuts.
5. Cover and cook for 4 hours on HIGH or 6 hours on LOW.

Nutritional information:

Calories 461

Total fat 28 g, saturated fat 5 g

Net carbohydrates 11 g

Protein 39 g

Rainy Day Bratwurst Pot

Cook Time: 4-6 hours
Prep Time: 10 minutes
Serves: 4

Ingredients:

1 pound bratwurst links, sliced thick
2 cups carrots, peeled and sliced
1 cup celery, sliced
1 cup red onion, diced
4 cups cabbage, sliced
2 cups chicken or vegetable stock
1 cup stewed tomatoes, with liquid
1 teaspoon thyme
1 teaspoon basil
1 teaspoon salt
1 teaspoon black pepper

Directions:

1. Set up and prepare your slow cooker.
2. Add the bratwurst along with the carrots, celery, red onion and cabbage.
3. Next add in the chicken or vegetable stock and the stewed tomatoes with the liquid.
4. Season with thyme, basil, salt and black pepper.
5. Cover and cook for 4 hours on HIGH, or 6 hours on LOW.

Nutritional information:

Calories 336
Total fat 23 g, saturated fat 8 g
Net carbohydrates 14 g
Protein 14 g

Curried Lamb

Cook Time: 4-6 hours
Prep Time: 10 minutes
Serves: 4

Ingredients:

1 pound lamb, cut into strips
1 cup apple, chopped
1 cup green bell pepper
½ cup celery, diced
2 cups broccoli florets
2 cups fresh snow peas
1 cup chicken or vegetable stock
1 cup coconut milk
1 tablespoon green curry paste
1 teaspoon fresh grated ginger
¼ cup fresh mint chopped

Directions:

1. Set up and prepare the slow cooker.
2. Place the lamb in the slow cooker, followed by the apple, green bell pepper, celery. If possible add the broccoli, and snow peas in the last 30-45 minutes of cooking, otherwise add it at the same time..
3. In a bowl combine the chicken or vegetable stock, coconut milk, green curry paste, ginger, and mint. Mix well and add to the slow cooker.
4. Cover and cook for 4 hours on LOW, or 6 hours on HIGH.

Nutritional information:

Calories 339

Total fat 18 g, saturated fat 12 g

Net carbohydrates 13 g

Protein 28 g

Variety of Vegetables

Who says that low carb living needs to be heavy with meat? Vegetables can be the star of a low carb meal just as easily as any meat. All you need is to know which vegetables to use and how to bring out the best flavors. These unique vegetable dishes will help you do just that.

Mexican Mock Mac and Cheese

Cook Time: 2 hours
Prep Time: 10 minutes
Serves: 4-6

Ingredients:
1 large head cauliflower, cut into small florets
2 cloves garlic, crushed and minced
1 cup tomatoes, diced
1 cup Monterey jack cheese, shredded
1 cup Cotija cheese, crumbled
½ cup cream cheese
1 cup vegetable or chicken stock
1 cup heavy cream
2 teaspoons ancho chili powder
1 teaspoon cumin
¼ cup fresh cilantro, chopped
1 teaspoon salt
1 teaspoon black pepper

Directions:

1. Set up and prepare your slow cooker.
2. Add the cauliflower, garlic, tomatoes, and vegetable stock.
3. Cover and cook for 2 hours on HIGH.
4. In a bowl, combine the Monterey jack cheese, Cotija cheese, cream cheese, heavy cream, ancho chili powder, cumin, cilantro, salt, and black pepper. Mix well.
5. About half an hour before you are ready to eat, stir the cheese mixture into the slow cooker until evenly distributed.
6. Cover and continue cooking until heated through.

Nutritional information:

Calories 459
Total fat 40 g, saturated fat 24 g
Net carbohydrates 9 g
Protein 16 g

Creamy Cabbage Au Gratin

Cook Time: 2 hours
Prep Time: 10 minutes
Serves: 4

Ingredients:

4 cups cabbage, shredded
1 cup carrots, peeled and sliced thinly
½ cup scallions, sliced
½ cup vegetable stock
½ cup milk
1 egg, beaten
½ cup fontina cheese, shredded
½ cup Swiss cheese, shredded
¼ cup fresh parsley, chopped
2 tablespoons fresh chives, chopped
1 teaspoon salt
1 teaspoon black pepper

Directions:

1. Set up and prepare your slow cooker.
2. Mix the cabbage, carrots, scallions, vegetable stock, milk, and egg in the slow cooker.
3. Cover and cook on HIGH for 2 hours.
4. Half an hour before you are ready to eat, add the fontina cheese, Swiss cheese, parsley, chives, salt, and black pepper.
5. Cover and continue cooking until the cheese is melted.

Nutritional information:

Calories 227

Total fat 14 g, saturated fat 8 g,

Net carbohydrates 8 g

Protein 15 g

Rustic Squash Bake

Cook Time: 4 hours
Prep Time: 10 minutes
Serves: 6

Ingredients:

4 cups butternut squash, peeled and cubed
1 cup acorn squash, peeled and cubed
1 cup yellow onion, diced
1 cup bacon, cooked and crumbled (optional)
1 ½ cups vegetable stock
½ cup unsweetened apple juice
½ cup pecans, chopped
1 teaspoon thyme
1 teaspoon nutmeg
1 teaspoon salt
1 teaspoon black pepper

Directions:

1. Set up and prepare your slow cooker.
2. Add the butternut squash to the slow cooker, followed by the acorn squash, yellow onion and bacon.
3. Add in the vegetable stock and apple juice.
4. Next, add the pecans and season with thyme, nutmeg, salt and black pepper.
5. Cover and cook for 4 hours on LOW.

Nutritional information:

Calories 176
Total fat 9 g, saturated fat 1 g
Net carbohydrates 15 g
Protein 4 g

Spaghetti Squash with Mushrooms and Peppers

Cook Time: 4 hours
Prep Time: 10 minutes
Serves: 4-6

Ingredients:
4 cups spaghetti squash (insides only)
2 cloves garlic, crushed and minced
3 cups cremini mushrooms, halved or quartered
1 cup red bell pepper, diced
1 cup walnuts, chopped
2 cups vegetable stock
1 sprig fresh rosemary
1 tablespoon fresh dill, chopped
1 tablespoon fresh chives, chopped
1 teaspoon salt
1 teaspoon black pepper
½ cup goat cheese, crumbled

Directions:
1. Set up and prepare your slow cooker.
2. In the slow cooker, combine the spaghetti squash, garlic, cremini mushrooms, red bell pepper, and walnuts.
3. Next, add the vegetable stock and season with rosemary, dill, chives, salt and black pepper.
4. Cover and cook for 4 hours on LOW.
5. Half an hour before you are ready to eat, remove the lid and add the goat cheese and stir. Cover and continue cooking

Nutritional information:

Calories 334

Total fat 27 g, saturated fat 6 g

Net carbohydrates 13 g

Protein 13 g

Creamy Spinach and Artichoke Casserole

Cook Time: 4 hours
Prep Time: 10 minutes
Serves: 6

Ingredients:

12 cups fresh spinach, torn
2 cups artichoke hearts, quartered
1 cup red onion, diced
3 cloves garlic, crushed and minced
1 ½ cups vegetable stock
1 tablespoon butter, diced
1 teaspoon crushed red pepper flakes
1 tablespoon fresh dill, chopped
¼ cup fresh parsley, chopped
1 teaspoon salt
1 teaspoon white pepper
1 cup walnuts, chopped
1 cup sour cream
1 cup Swiss cheese, shredded
½ cup goat cheese, crumbled
¼ cup fresh grated Parmesan cheese

Directions:

1. Set up and prepare your slow cooker.
2. In the slow cooker, mix the artichoke hearts, red onion, garlic, vegetable stock, and butter.
3. Season with the crushed red pepper flakes, dill, parsley, salt and white pepper.
4. Cover and cook on LOW for 4 hours.

5. Half an hour before you are ready to eat, remove the lid and add the spinach, walnuts, sour cream, Swiss cheese, goat cheese, and Parmesan. Mix until well blended.
6. Cover and continue cooking until ready to serve.

Nutritional information:
Calories 388
Total fat 32 g, saturated fat 13 g
Net carbohydrates 11 g
Protein 15 g

Slow Cooked Ratatouille

Cook Time: 4 hours
Prep Time: 10 minutes
Serves: 4-6

Ingredients:
2 cups canned tomatoes, with liquid
3 tablespoons tomato paste
1 ½ cups vegetable stock
3 cloves garlic, crushed and minced
4 cups eggplant, peeled and cubed
4 cups zucchini, sliced
2 cups summer squash, peeled and sliced
1 cup green bell pepper, diced
1 cup red onion, diced
2 teaspoons Italian seasoning
1 teaspoon onion powder
1 teaspoon salt
1 teaspoon black pepper

Directions:
1. Set up and prepare your slow cooker.
2. In the slow cooker, combine the canned tomatoes with liquid, tomato paste, and vegetable stock.
3. Add the garlic, eggplant, zucchini, summer squash, green bell pepper, and onion.
4. Season with the Italian seasoning, onion powder, salt, and black pepper.
5. Cover and cook on LOW for 4 hours.

Nutritional information:

Calories 119

Total fat 1 g, saturated fat 0 g

Net carbohydrates 15 g

Protein 5 g

Green Bean and Mushroom Casserole

Cook Time: 4 hours
Prep Time: 10 minutes
Serves: 6

Ingredients:

8 cups fresh green beans, trimmed
2 cups fresh mushrooms, sliced
1 cup water chestnuts, drained and chopped
1 cup yellow onion, diced
2 tablespoons butter, diced
1 ½ cups vegetable stock
1 tablespoon soy sauce
1 teaspoon crushed red pepper flakes
1 tablespoon fresh chives, chopped
1 teaspoon garlic powder
¼ cup fresh parsley, chopped
1 cup sour cream
½ cup heavy cream
½ cup Parmesan cheese
Sliced almonds, for garnish if desired

Directions:

1. Set up and prepare your slow cooker.
2. In the slow cooker combine, the green beans, mushrooms, water chestnuts, yellow onion, and butter. Toss to mix.
3. In a bowl, combine the vegetable stock, soy sauce, crushed red pepper flakes, chives, and garlic powder.
4. Cover and cook on LOW for 4 hours.
5. Half an hour before you are ready to eat, remove the lid and stir in the parsley, sour cream, heavy

cream, and Parmesan. Continue cooking until heated through.

6. Serve garnished with almond sliced.

Nutritional information:

Calories 307

Total fat 22 g, saturated fat 14 g

Net carbohydrates 15 g

Protein 9 g

Conclusion

We know that the use of a slow cooker offers countless benefits in terms of meal options and healthy food choices. In general, using a slow cooker saves time and energy, giving you more time to devote to all of the other aspects of your life. But sometimes, with certain dietary considerations, the use of a slow cooker seems ineffective or even cumbersome. The purpose of this book has been to show you that when it comes to low carb eating, the slow cooker is definitely your friend on the path to great health.

With fresh, wholesome ingredients, there is no limit to the culinary delights that you can create in your slow cooker. This book is merely a starting point to provide you with the inspiration to truly embrace low carb living and make every day and every meal as exciting as possible for a lifetime of good health and good eating.

About the author

Sarah Spencer, who lives in Canada with her husband and two children, describes herself as an avid foodie who prefers watching the Food Network over a hockey game or NCIS! She is a passionate cook who dedicates all her time between creating new recipes, writing cookbooks, and her family, though not necessarily in that order!

Sarah has had two major influences in her life regarding cooking, her Grandmother and Mama Li.

She was introduced to cooking at an early age by her Grandmother who thought cooking for your loved ones was the single most important thing in life. Not only that, but she was the World's Best Cook in the eyes of all those lucky enough to taste her well-kept secret recipes. Over the years, she conveyed her knowledge and appreciation of food to Sarah.

Sarah moved to Philadelphia when her father was transferred there when Sarah was a young teenager. She became close friends with a girl named Jade, whose parents owned a Chinese take-out restaurant. This is when Sarah met her second biggest influence,

Mama Li. Mama Li was Jade's mother and a professional cook in her own restaurant. Sarah would spend many hours in the restaurant as a helper to Mama Li. Her first job was in the restaurant. Mama Li showed Sarah all about cooking Asian food, knife handling, and mixing just the right amount of spices. Sarah became an excellent Asian cook, especially in Chinese and Thai food.

Along the way, Sarah developed her own style in the kitchen. She loves to try new flavors and mix up ingredients in new and innovative ways. She is also very sensitive to her son's allergy to gluten and has been cooking gluten-free and paleo recipes for quite some time.

More Books from Sarah Spencer

Shown below are some of her other books. To check any of them out, just click on the book cover you like. Follow Sarah and join in her great love of cooking!

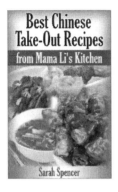
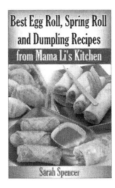
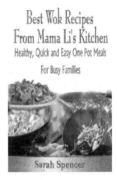

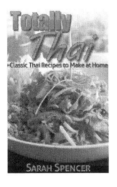
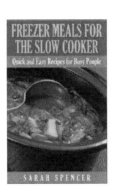
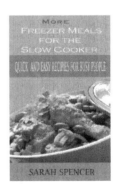

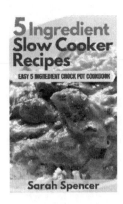

5 Ingredient Slow Cooker Recipes
EASY 5 INGREDIENT CROCK POT COOKBOOK
Sarah Spencer

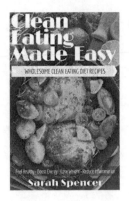

Clean Eating Made Easy
WHOLESOME CLEAN EATING DIET RECIPES
Feel Healthy · Boost Energy · Lose Weight · Reduce Inflammation
Sarah Spencer

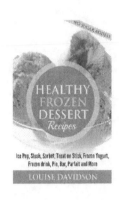

NO SUGAR ADDED
HEALTHY FROZEN DESSERT Recipes
Ice Pop, Slush, Sorbet, Treat on Stick, Frozen Yogurt, Frozen drink, Pie, Bar, Parfait and More
LOUISE DAVIDSON

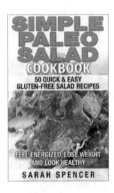

SIMPLE PALEO SALAD COOKBOOK
50 QUICK & EASY GLUTEN-FREE SALAD RECIPES
FEEL ENERGIZED, LOSE WEIGHT AND LOOK HEALTHY
SARAH SPENCER

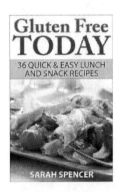

Gluten Free TODAY
36 QUICK & EASY LUNCH AND SNACK RECIPES
SARAH SPENCER

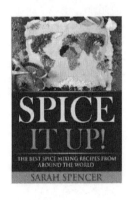

SPICE IT UP!
THE BEST SPICE MIXING RECIPES FROM AROUND THE WORLD
SARAH SPENCER

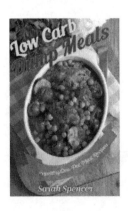

Low Carb Dump Meals
Sarah Spencer

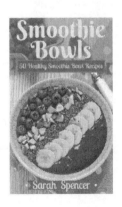

Smoothie Bowls
50 Healthy Smoothie Bowl Recipes
· Sarah Spencer ·

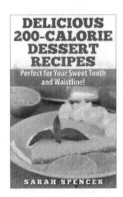

DELICIOUS 200-CALORIE DESSERT RECIPES
Perfect for Your Sweet Tooth and Waistline!
SARAH SPENCER